HCG DIET

Table of Contents

DISCLAIMER

The information contained within this document is intended for informative and not prescriptive use. Follow the advice of your doctor when considering a change in diet or beginning an exercise routine. While we strive to provide accurate information and ensure a healthy, successful plan, all bodies are different and will react to different diets and exercises in different ways. If you intend to follow the diet and exercise tips contained in this document, and you aren't sure if they will adversely affect your health, it is highly recommended that you speak with your regular doctor or with a nutritionist before beginning any program associated with this document.

Introduction

I want to thank you and congratulate you for downloading the book, *"HCG DIET"*

This book contains proven steps and strategies on how to lose weight.

The HCG diet exists as a body mass loss procedure that helps overweight folks to drop an average of two pounds each day. A 500 calorie daily diet, likewise known by way of a very little calorie diet or VLCD, stays combined by a marginal HCG intake.

A usual hormone that remains created at laboratories, HCG raises the metabolic rate of the body while utilizing stored lipids for dynamism. The consequence of this is a significant fat loss in an extremely short period.

There exist numerous HCG protocols for losing weight. HCG weight loss shots; However, are not yet approved for losing weight by the Food and Drug Administration. Nonetheless, it works where other food regimens fail. Bear in mind that everyone owns a customary calorie number where their physique burns at a day today basis. This figure is established by the weight, sexual category, height, dimensions, and regular activities of any person.

The regular person could have an average rate of burning or metabolism of 2,450 each day. Moreover, this number changes once food consumption changes. When you alter your consumption to a lower amount, your physique reprograms its figures to suit those alterations. Say your physique has a figure of 2000. This implies that with your dimension and activity, besides food consumption, your physique burns around 2000 calories each day. On the assumption that this remains constant, you will not see any change within your body mass, but, if suddenly, you lessen your consumption, your physique burns whatsoever it can to satisfy its requirements and that is why people lose body mass.

What is bad happens when your physique can become careless in burning and that it burns muscles and vital fats in place of unhealthy stowed fat. On the other hand, when you raise your consumption, your physique takes what is left as soon as it uses its metabolic rate figure and keeps the excess for later days. Some individuals might use it on the following day when they possess surplus metabolism available or maybe when they did not eat the same quantity on the subsequent day where the body needs more.

This book will teach you how you can motivate yourself to be the healthier version of yourself. If becoming healthy is not enough to motivate you, this book will help you realize just how much you can gain when you reach your target weight.

This book should serve as your diet buddy all throughout your HCG diet plan journey. It has everything you need to know about the HCG treatment, the challenges, and how you can get past through those challenges.

This book will also serve as your guide as to how you can maintain your ideal weight once you are already there. There will be tips and life-changing realizations that you can learn by reading this book.

Thanks again for downloading this book, I hope you enjoy it!

This document is geared towards providing exact and reliable information in regards to the topic and issue covered. The publication is sold with the idea that the publisher is not required to render accounting, officially permitted, or otherwise, qualified services. If advice is necessary, legal or professional, a practiced individual in the profession should be ordered.

- From a Declaration of Principles which was accepted and approved equally by a Committee of the American Bar Association and a Committee of Publishers and Associations.

In no way is it legal to reproduce, duplicate, or transmit any part of this document in either electronic means or in printed format. Recording of this publication is strictly prohibited and any storage of this document is not allowed unless with written permission from the publisher. All rights reserved.

The information provided herein is stated to be truthful and consistent, in that any liability, in terms of inattention or otherwise, by any usage or abuse of any policies, processes, or directions contained within is the solitary and utter responsibility of the recipient reader. Under no circumstances will any legal responsibility or blame be held against the publisher for any reparation, damages, or monetary loss due to the information herein, either directly or indirectly.

Respective authors own all copyrights not held by the publisher.

The information herein is offered for informational purposes solely, and is universal as so. The presentation of the information is without contract or any type of guarantee assurance.

The trademarks that are used are without any consent, and the publication of the trademark is without permission or backing by the trademark owner. All trademarks and brands within this book are for clarifying purposes only and are the owned by the owners themselves, not affiliated with this document.

Chapter 1 - What is a HCG diet?

On the HCG diet, individuals are able to lose a significant amount of weight without a lot of exercise. Moreover, this weight comes off fast. Those who have been on the diet claim they have lost up to 40 pounds in 40 days. Keeping this in mind, it is important to know that to do it, you will need to have the HCG drops or injections, which may be available through your doctor or purchased online.

You should have the confidence to start with the HCG diet plan as you are now well-equipped with all the knowledge and motivation necessary to start the plan. If in any stage of the program you feel like doubting yourself, feel free to pick this book up again and read it so you can have a reminder why you are doing what you are doing. You should have this book on your entire journey so you will not have a chance to doubt whether what you are doing is beneficial for you.

Being overweight is not healthy. And by following the HCG diet plan, you are on your way to a healthier you and you can be there fast.

Once you have them, the guidelines are clear. During the initial phase, you will eat no more than 500 calories per day. During that phase, the goal is to eat what your body needs but still lose weight. You will also not feel hungry on this plan.

H CG is a short form for Human Chorionic Gonadotrophin. This hormone is produced by women during early stages of their pregnancy. Studies have revealed that a small, daily intake of HCG supplement will result in weight loss for most healthy people. The weight loss through HCG is normally around 1-2 lbs a day, and often more, when accompanied with very low calorie diet (VLCD).

The HCG diet contains three phases. The HCG Diet phases are:

Phase 1 Loading— two days of eating fatty and carbfilled foods.

Phase 2 Burning— 2643 days of 500 calorie diet, depending on your goal.

Phase 3 Maintenance— 3 weeks of a sugar/starch free diet.

The loading phase requires that we begin taking HCG and load ourselves with foods that are high in fats and carbohydrates. This is done with the intention that our body will start to adapt to effects of HCG. In the burning phase, we begin VLCD while continuing with drops. The maintenance phase requires that we not eat any starches or sugar for a specified time period

This diet plan is divided into three phases that help promote weight loss in the healthiest way.

The three phases are as follows:

1) Phase 1

Phase 1 of the HCG diet program requires weightwatchers or dieters to eat as much as food as they want, especially foods loaded with fat. This is intended for generating a store of fat to fight against headaches or hunger pangs that may develop after passing through the low-cal phase. In this phase, weight watchers or dieters should begin injecting HCG hormones into their body. It normally takes two days for this hormone to be absorbed into our system.

2) Phase 2

Phase 2 of the HCG diet is the most important phase. You must set a weight goal in your mind. This second phase normally lasts between 26 to 42 days. Unlike Phase 1, this part of HCG diet requires followers to follow the HCG meal plan strictly. The HCG diet plan is very food specific, particularly on the amount that should be consumed and digested by our body. The program requires us to consume only 500 calories per day on a low-carb, high-protein meal plan. The HCG injections also continue for the same period except for the last three days of the HCG diet. During those days, weight watchers should continue the meal plan but stop HCG injections.

3) HCG diet phase 3

Phase 3, the final phase of the HCG diet, is called the maintenance phase. This is one of the most important phases in HCG diet. When you reach the last day of your HCG diet, you must stay on the 500 calorie diet for three more days. This will make sure that all the HCG traces are out of our system before we start to introduce larger portions of foods back into our body.

Before returning to a normal diet, you must follow this phase to help your body adapt to other foods. For next three weeks, you must not eat any sugars or starches; otherwise you may start to return to a normal diet. Your body needs this much time to stabilize, so when three weeks pass, you should reintroduce foods into our diet. When you are near the end of this maintenance phase, you should slowly introduce starches and sugars into your diet.

In this phase you should keep an eye on your weight and record your weight each morning and stay within two lbs of the ideal weight. If you gain more than two lbs in any given day, you should skip a meal. This will help our body regulate your appetite and your weight.

The road to weight loss is not always easy. You should always bear in mind the goals that you want to achieve so you develop self-control and discipline. You will surely be on your way to healthy weight loss.

Why Do You Need To Be In This Diet Plan?

People who have used the HCG diet plan have made tremendous improvements in terms of the weighing scale. You can lose as much as one pound a day by sticking to the diet plan. Although the results may vary depending on the body mass and structure, you should see some improvement in as little as one week. You just have to see it for yourself and start the plan right away.

After weeks of following the diet plan, you should see a better change than you ever thought was possible. You can drastically change your future as you have gained a new-found confidence to face just about anything. Your confidence will stem from the fact that you have become a better version of yourself.

You will find more opportunities to be in any role you want; be it in a highly-competitive office, in the social scene, or having your own business. You will not have to catch your breath when going up a flight of stairs or drag yourself toward your destination because of the excess weight.

For some, there is a deep-seated motivation as to why they want to lose weight. You might be one of those who have always been bullied because you are overweight. You might have lost some career and life opportunities because of your weight. It is a known fact that obese people are being judged and discriminated in our society. You can change that by being healthier and leading a healthy lifestyle.

To be fully engaged in the HCG diet plan, you need to find your own motivation. If being healthier is not enough of a motivation, search deep within you so you will have the courage to stay in the diet plan no matter how hard it turns out to be. The first few weeks are the hardest and this is when it is easiest to quit. Find that motivation and hold on to it even after you have reached your goal. If you think getting to your desired weight is hard, maintaining it is even harder.

But if you have hard-wired yourself that you want to be this person, then you should be able to get through it.

All throughout the process, you need to stay positive even if you do not lose at the same pace with other people. What is important is that you are seeing improvements, no matter how small they may be. It is not good to pit yourself with other people; this is your journey after all.

Every time you weigh yourself and see an improvement, you should be proud of yourself. You have worked so hard to be where you are and it should not be too long before you reach your desired weight. You need to understand that every person's body adapt and react in different ways. If you are strictly following the diet plan, then you are not doing anything wrong. It is just the way your body is adapting and reacting to the change in your lifestyle.

Chapter 2 - how the diet works

For two days, you will eat as many high calorie foods and high fat foods as you like. You will take the drops for these two days.

For the next 23 days, you will take the drops and you will consume a low-calorie diet.

For the next three days, you continue to eat on the diet plan but you do not take drops.

If you follow this plan, you can lose a substantial amount of weight in a short period of time.

How does it work? In short, the creator of this plan found that by injecting HCG, which is a hormone produced by the body during pregnancy, it helps to accelerate weight loss by working to suppress the appetite. In addition, it works to blast away fat in the process.

A.T.W. Simeons is the creator of the diet and in his book, "Pounds and Inches: A New Approach to Obesity" he outlines the diet fully.

Today, there are dozens of message boards and resources all aimed at helping individuals to make it through this diet. What is astonishing is that so many people find it to be successful and easy to do. Many of them did not think they could be successful at this plan, but after working through the initial phases, they learned quickly that the weight was coming right off.

To be successful, you will need to follow a strict set of guidelines in which the following rules apply:

- 100 to 125 ounces of meat, including beef, chicken breast, white fish, lobster, crab, shrimp or turkey (no fatty content)

- 100 ounces of vegetables including spinach, chicory, onions, fennel, celery, tomatoes, green salad, cabbage, beets, red radishes, cucumbers and chard
- 1 breadstick or Melba toast serving
- An apple, orange, grapefruit or six to nine strawberries

If you can do this, you may find yourself with a fantastic diet plan that can help you to achieve every one of your health goals. To make it easier for you, we have broken the process down and provided you with some great tips and recipes included on the following pages.

Some diet plans just aim at reducing people's body weight. The real challenge is whether or not they have the capacity to maintain the body weight in long run. This is what is good about HCG diet. We will be able to sustain our body weight even if this diet plan ends. This is possible because HCG diet acts like a double action approach. The primary goal of this diet is to reduce fat in central parts of human body, the secondary goal of this diet focuses on maintenance of body weight the moment the diet plan's period completes. So by doing maintenance phase of HCG diet we'll be able to find out which foods work for us and which don't, allowing us to make long-lasting changes which will keep off the weight forever.

The reason that makes it possible is that energy needed by a person for her or his survival is diverted from the collected fat in various parts of body. Apart from these advantages, the HCG diet is relatively low cost and there are no mandatory foods, pills, fads, or any other type of weight loss treatment that people must follow.

There are two ways to ingest HCG hormone. It can be given through injections or orally. The HCG diet is combined with a low-calorie diet helps with improving body's metabolism naturally, which consequently allows the body to discard fat from hips, buttocks, thighs, abdomen, and neckline with ease. However, HCG drops are far safer than injections. And many HCG followers prefer to take it orally rather than inject it into their body.

Mindset Preparation

If you are one of those who have always been overweight their entire life or you simply want to lose the excess weight that you have gained over the past months, then here is a diet regimen that just might work for you. The HCG diet plan will allow you to lose the extra fat, and you will lose it fast. It may seem too far-fetched, but now, it is possible. By following a rigorous diet plan and taking the HCG supplement, you should be at your ideal weight in no time.

But first, let us go over the basics. HCG stands for human chorionic gonadotropin. It is the hormone produced during pregnancy that impedes a pregnant woman's feeling of hunger. By taking an HCG supplement, your body will respond the same way. You will not feel hungry right away and you will want smaller portions of food.

The hormone may also promote fat loss. Along with the HCG supplement, you will need to follow a very strict diet of 500 calories a day. This may seem like a small average – a person needing at least 2000 calories daily. But the 500 calories a day is only during the first few days, at the time when you just have to burn the excess fats on your body. Once you are past this stage, you can gradually increase your calorie intake as described in the next chapters.

Before you jump into this diet plan, you will need to have a strong motivation connected to why you have to lose the extra weight. Early on, you need to know that strictly adhering to the diet plan may prove to be tough. You will have to go through a serious change in your lifestyle that other people may find too difficult to follow. That is why you need to draw a clear picture of who you want to be before you start. And from there, you must use that to motivate yourself until you become that person.

Aside from the aesthetic benefits of following the diet plan, you also need to remember that being overweight is not healthy; not only physically, but mentally and emotionally as well. A lot of overweight people have to go through every day of their lives not liking the person they see on the mirror. If you are one of them, then it is time for you to take charge.

You need to know that it is possible to lose weight by following the diet, and maintain a healthy lifestyle. It is time to ditch the old mentality that you are just born fat and that there is nothing you can do about it. This is your body we are talking about and there is certainly something you can do.

To set your expectation, the road to achieving your ideal body may not be easy. This is the case for every diet plan there is. But the rewards of your hardships will be all worth it. As Sophocles once said, "There is no success without hardship." So to be that person you have illustrated on your mind, you have to work hard and follow the diet plan to a T.

Chapter 3 - Benefits of HCG diet

1. Loose Skin:

HCG drops are currently enormously well known in the weight reduction hover for producing incredible weight decrease comes about when utilized alongside a low calorie consume less calories.

This benefit of HCG drops have been tested in weight reduction trials and has turned out to be a protected and successful approach to get more fit.

This is a hormone actually delivered amid pregnancy. Individuals taking HCG procedure consume less calories commonly get HCG infusions. HCG tabs is an option. People eating less carbs because of HCG has extremely confines calories to approximately few hundreds calories a daily. That is just percent quarter of the around few thousand calories the normal grown-up requires daily, as indicated by the Doctors online. Fast weight reduction that can happen with HCG eat less carbs and other with reduction arrangements can affect the skin.

2. Essential Weight Lost

The normal HCG calorie counter ordinarily reduce two lb daily sometimes over 30 lb monthly. Skin could be overly distressed due to excess elasticity and neglect to withdraw and fix after a considerable weight reduction, Body has a tendency to lose versatility as it has extended for a longer time frame. Accordingly, abundance skin seems free and droopy.

Impacts: Individuals that shed weight of an hundred lb. on the other hand may wind up with considerable measures of substantial and abundance flesh around their face and around the trunk, rump, belly, torso hand and hips. Their level of sagginess can differ contingent upon your age, nature of body, skin and quantity of lbs lost.

3. HCG Prevent Occurrence:

Cancer prevention agents rich nourishment, for example blueberries,nuts spinach, salmon, carrots and tomatoes seem to possess a defensive impact for body. Be that as it may, the hospitals brings up it is practically impossible to just "tone up" a lot of free skin flesh unless it is surgically evacuated using Skin Countering procedure.

4. No Surgery

Simple non-surgical method might be used now and again to fix free skin taking after quick weight reduction through Liposuction . Laser revival may unassumingly fix free facial skin, takes note of the school of Dermatology and Body Care (AAD) . A cosmetic touch up will normally have all the more significantly and longer enduring outcomes i.e facial lift

These benefits are the more reasons why my people interested in weight loss embrace HCG.

Being smart in pretty skin has a lot of advantages. Fit appearances in social gatherings is attractive. Clothes fits better on the body usually a great smile can complement that.

Movie roles for ideal beauty and being sexy is an advantage for individuals who are Actress.

Chapter 4 - Possible side-effects of HCG diet plan

Constipation

We'll be eating a lot less than we're used to, and obviously there will be less to excrete. People on HCG diet may have bowel movements as much as three to four days apart. This is not considered true constipation unless you know you need to go but cannot. A mild laxative (sugar-free) will solve these troubles. You should also drink plenty of water to help smooth out your tract and soften up stool.

Headache

During first week of HCG diet our body has to adjust, and you may experience headaches. This one probably is the most usual side effect. You can take any over-the-counter painkillers to treat this trouble. Also make sure to drink lots of water every day during the HCG diet.

Dizziness

Another quite common, but temporary, side effect of this low-carb, low-calorie HCG diet plan is dizziness. It is usually mild and almost goes away after the first week.

Leg Cramps

This is one rare side effect that is caused by low potassium levels you will get on HCG diet. It can be easily treated by taking a supplement of potassium. Taking a multivitamin could be even better (like Vita-X).

Rash

Another rare side effect is skin rash. On HCG diet, our body will burn and consume fat at an unbelievable speed. When fat cells are consumed, normal toxins will be released into body. If those toxins build up, they are likely to cause skin rash. This trouble can be reduced by drinking a lot of water to help flush those toxins out.

Hair Thinning

Some weight watchers report the problem of hair thinning. If it happens at all, it will be temporary. Normally, hair thinning, if it happens, begins after three months of dieting continuously. If it happens you should increase your intake of protein.

The above mentioned side effects only occur in a small section of HCG followers, and as stated earlier it can often be prevented and treated with very common medicines.

Other Concerns

Some concerns from a VLCD (very low calorie diet) may include heart issues such as palpitations or arrhythmias and gallstone formation.

Heart issues are obviously a more concerning issue and it needs to be dealt with. The reality is that VLCD programs have not been proven to be the cause of reported heart issues.

However, with gallstones, it takes a few or more months of continuous dieting for a 12% -25% chances of forming them, and they are usually small. In other words HCG diet is extremely unlikely to cause any problems there.

As always, if you experience any symptoms that concern you during the diet—unusual anxieties or pains or just have a bad experience— you should stop this diet and check with any medical professional. This diet is not meant for pregnant women, breastfeeding women, children, or anyone with a pre-existing medical condition. The key fact to be remembered here is that we are on diet just for a few weeks; it is not for a lifetime.

Chapter 5 - Food List for HCG Diet

This is a list of foods you can eat while doing HCG Diet

Phase 2.

Use this list as a quick reference guide for shopping and preparing HCG Diet meals.

Vegetables

- Any type of lettuce, beet greens, spinach, chard, cabbage
- Any type of tomatoes
- Any type of onions
- Fennel
- Cucumber
- Asparagus
- Celery
- Radishes

Proteins

- All meats have to be trimmed of all fat (and skin)
- White Fish
- Crab
- Lobster
- Shrimp
- Chicken
- Extra Lean Beef (steak, 96% lean ground beef, pot roast)

Fruit

- Apples

- Lemons
- Blackberries, blueberries, or strawberries

Drinks & Others

- Herbal Tea
- Melba Toast
- Sugarless Gum
- Bottled Water
- Stevia (natural sweetener, any flavour)
- Braggs Liquid Amino (a type of soy sauce)
- Apple Cider Vinegar
- Mustard
- Any natural herbs or spices, garlic, salt, and pepper

Quick and Helpful Tips for HCG Diet:

- We should measure ourselves and weight ourselves before we start.
- We should take a before photograph.
- We should spread our food intake throughout the day; it will lessen our hunger so we are not as likely to overeat.
- We should plenty of drink water, it helps flush out the fat.
- We should pre-plan our meals; if we come home hungry we are more likely to go off the diet if we don't have our meal planned. We should get a good recipe book.
- We should stay focused on our goal: good health at a good weight.
- We should drink water; it helps with potential constipation.
- We should learn to prepare easy and quick five minute meals.

- We should not use oil-based cosmetics, oil-based body care or oil-based skin care. We should use only water-based skin and body care products.
- We should drink plenty of water to keep our body and skin well hydrated.
- We should meditate or pray to keep ourselves focused.
- We should buy clothes at thrift store until we reach our weight goal, and then we can have a shopping spree.
- We should sign up for any HCG news groups for doses of support.
- We should take time for ourselves.
- If we do get hungry, we should drink some more water and add another meal in our day as a treat.
- If we get stuck at the same weight for some days, we should do the "eat apples all day" trick for a jumpstart. If that does not help, we should go on maintenance phase for a couple of weeks.

Chapter 6 - How to Track Your Weekly Progress

During the first few weeks of the HCG diet plan, it is important to track your weekly progress. You can easily feel discouraged if your body does not show any sign of improvement. However, not until you step into a weighing scale will you know that there is actually an improvement. The physical improvements will not be visible right away. You have to stay patient and track your weekly progress so you will stay motivated. Aside from the motivations you have outlined in Chapters 1 and 2, your weekly progress should be a form of motivation in itself.

You can use the weight chart at the end of this book to track your weekly progress. Writing down your progress will give you a better feel of how you are doing. You can actually compare your data week after week and use those improvements to further your journey.

You should also take progress pictures. Start with right before you start the HCG diet plan until you reach your target weight. A visual reminder of how you were before and where you are right now should be a motivating factor for you to keep on pushing.

You will also need to buy a weighing scale and use it weekly so you will see how you tip the scale. Your weighing scale should be your diet buddy that can give you unbiased and accurate answers to whether you are losing weight or not. A weighing scale is essential in tracking your progress. Without a weighing scale, you will just have to guess how you are doing.

Aside from the motivating factors provided by tracking your progress, you will also know whether the plan is working for you.

You may feel skeptical at first, especially when there are no visible improvements. But if you have a written and photographic evidence of how you are doing, then you will know every inch of improvement that you are going through.

You can even use your progress as proof so you can help other people who also want to lose weight. Some people need hard evidence before they believe anything to be true, and this is not a bad thing at all. You also need to practice the same thing so you will not get trapped into a diet plan that does not work for you.

Our bodies work in different ways. Another person's body may respond positively to a specific diet plan while others do not. While some diet plans are not really designed to work, some may offer great results. You should totally skip the diet plans that do not work. The trick is finding the plan that actually works and ensuring that it will work on you. The only way to know for sure is by tracking your progress. You should also keep tabs of what you can do more so you can get to your desired weight in the least amount of time without sacrificing your health.

Getting Through the HCG Diet

As with any other diet plan, there are the challenging parts. These are the times when you feel that you are doing so much but producing very little results. But most people quit right after they started.

For one, the early days are usually the hardest part. This is when you have to make changes and changes do come very hard. And once you feel that challenge, you may tend to quit right away thinking that you have not invested that much anyway, so it's okay to give up.

The thing is, it is not okay. It is not okay to live throughout your life feeling defeated. To think that there is nothing you can do is unacceptable. You have to dig deep and decide that you want to change your life. You can change your destiny by sticking to what you really want instead of settling to what is comfortable for you.

As with the HCG diet plan, the hardest part is sticking to a strict calorie limit. Food is readily available for you; your instinct is to grab that food and have a bite. If you intend to go through the HCG diet plan, the food mentality of grab and go will not work. You have to follow the diet described in Chapter 3 to achieve the results that you want. You should not worry about feeling hungry, as the HCG hormone will help you to not feel the hunger.

For the HCG diet plan to work, you need to strictly follow all the procedures. If necessary, you may need to admit yourself in the clinic where your shots will be administered. This is to ensure that you are given the shots you need and that your food is prepared the way it should be and in the right amount. You do not have to be confined in the hospital all day. You are allowed to leave and stroll around as long as you do not consume food while you are out of the hospital. Nevertheless, it is also perfectly fine to be an outpatient, given that you have the strength and motivation to stick to the plan despite all the food around you.

You do not have to be in the 500 calorie diet all throughout. After finishing the diet plan, you can resume to regular eating as long as you restrict your intake of starch and sugar.

During the course of your treatment with HCG, you will not be required to work out because the low calorie diet will have to use the stored fats in your body for energy. However, after the treatment, you can work out to reduce the appearance of sagging skin. You can start to build muscles after you have achieved your ideal weight. Working out is also a good way to burn up calories since you would have resumed to regular eating by then. This will also aid in maintaining your weight so you will not feel like a failure once your weight goes up again.

After the HCG treatment, it is up to you to take care of yourself. And taking of yourself includes watching what you eat and working out.

Chapter 7 - Post-HCG Diet Plan

After you have achieved your ideal weight, one of the challenges of being in the post HCG diet plan is knowing how to move forward. After the HCG diet plan, you will be allowed to have regular portions of food. You should not be overly excited about this and begin eating everything that you want. You should remember that the reason you were overweight before is because of your poor eating habits. You should not over-indulge thinking that your body will not go back to where it was before. It is an ever-looming possibility especially if you do not take good measures to maintain your weight.

After the HCG diet plan, you should be more conscious with what you eat. You should follow a low-fat diet and limit your consumption of starchy foods and sugar. You can also start to work out so you can have a more toned and healthy body. One of the main reasons that your body stores up fat is that the sugars you consume are not converted into energy. By working out, you are enabling your body to use up calories and any excess fat so they do not get stored in your body-which could eventually cause obesity.

Being overweight should be a thing in the past for you once you reach this stage. You should be more motivated to keep your body because you worked hard for it and you deserve it. Do not let all your hard work go to waste by neglecting your body and forgetting what the HCG diet plan has taught you.

Having a healthy body is a product of a healthy lifestyle. Everything that you put in your mouth will be reflected in your figure and in the weighing scale so you need to choose well and choose right. You should not consume foods that are not needed by your body. Eat right and eat when you have to. You should know by now how you can interpret your body's needs. There is no need to eat when you are not hungry. You need to remove the habit of binge eating as it adds to much of your weight.

You should eat to nourish your body. Eating should not be a means to cure your boredom or to manage your emotions. You need to find other ways to pass the time.

You can start to pick up a hobby and become busy so you can take your mind off from eating unnecessarily. You may also need to find other ways to manage your stress and emotions. Being an emotional eater is not healthy as you tend to consume more food to make yourself feel better. The reality here is that overeating will not take all your problems away. And overeating may impose another problem for you.

Ultimately, having a healthy body solves a myriad of things for you. You get to enjoy the tangible benefits of having a great figure. Aside from that, you get to love yourself more and have the feeling that you are in charge. You are healthy physically, mentally, and emotionally.

Your Weight Loss Chart And Journal

Instructions in using the weight loss chart

Materials:

For the weight loss chart, you will need the chart, a weighing scale, a pen, and lots of motivation and perseverance.

Procedures:

1. Fill in the month's column. Write what month of the year it is so you will know when you started and you can have a record of your monthly progress.

2. Under the Week Column, you should write the week number that you are currently in. You should record your

week number at the end of every week. Your first entry should be Week 0. Your next entry will be Week 1 and that is 7 days after you recorded your initial weight.

3. On the Weight Column, you should write the weight registered on your weighing scale at the end of every week. Your first entry should be your weight prior to starting the diet plan. The next entry will be your weight at the end of the following weeks.

4. The Goal Weight Column should contain your target weight at the end of every week. Do not create goals that are too high or too low. You need the right amount of motivation to keep you afloat. Setting a goal that is too high may dampen your spirit especially when you are not meeting them week after week. But setting a goal that is too low may also set the wrong expectations. When setting your goal, you must be realistic.

5. Under the Goal Met? Column, you just need to write if your weight at the end of the week matches you goal weight. This is just a Yes and No Column.

6. Under the Notes, you will need to write your observations every week and deviations from the diet plan, if any. You can also note the difference in your weight and goal weight to see how far you are from where you want to be in a weekly basis. You can also write your progress as compared with the previous week under the Notes Column.

Chapter 8 - HCG Diet recipes

Breakfast

Simple Coleslaw

- 3 ½ oz. cabbage, shredded
- Vinegar
- Basil, rosemary and cumin
- Salt
- Mix cabbage with vinegar and spices to taste. Serve immediately.

Apple Cuke Salad

- 1 cucumber, sliced
- ½ apple, chopped
- 1 Tblsp. water
- 2 Tblsp. apple cider vinegar
- Garlic salt
- Pepper
- Toss cucumber and apple together. In a jar, shake the remaining ingredients and pour over the salad. You can add a little stevia if desired, for sweetness.

Cucumber Salad

- ½ cucumber, sliced
- 1 Tblsp. vinegar

- 1 tsp. dill
- ½ tsp. stevia
- Pepper
- Mix dill, stevia, pepper and vinegar together. Toss with cucumbers and refrigerate for at least 2 hours or overnight.

Broccoli Slaw

- ½ head of broccoli, grated
- ¼ c. carrot, grated
- ¼ c. red cabbage, grated
- Toss all ingredients with 2 Tblsp. of dressing of your choice.

Garlic Greens

- 2 c. greens of your choice
- ¼ c. vegetable broth
- 3 cloves garlic, minced
- ¼ tsp. red pepper flakes
- 2 Tblsp. onion, chopped
- 4 Tblsp. lemon juice
- Salt
- Bring broth (can substitute water) to a boil in a medium pot along with garlic, onion and spices.
- Add the greens and cook, covered for 15 minutes.
- Season with lemon and salt to taste.

Lemon Spinach Soup

- 2 c. vegetable broth
- 2 tsp. lemon juice

- 1 lb. spinach
- ½ tsp. thyme
- Salt to taste
- Put lemon juice, broth and thyme, along with salt, into a pot and bring to a boil.
- Place the spinach in bowls and pour the boiling soup over them for a tasty soup.

Asparagus Soup

- 1/4 lb. asparagus
- 1/4 c. low sodium chicken broth
- 1/8 tsp. garlic powder
- Salt and pepper
- Cook all ingredients over medium high heat until asparagus is tender.
- Blend in blender until smooth and serve warm.

Spinach Chips

- 1 lb. fresh spinach
- Juice of one lemon
- Salt
- Mix salt and juice together until salt dissolves. Lay spinach leaves in a dehydrator and spritz with the lemon mixture. Dehydrate until crispy.

Creole Cucumbers

- 2 c. cucumber, sliced
- 1/8 tsp. creole seasoning

- Toss seasoning and cucumbers together for a spicy side dish.

Caramelized Onions

- 1 large sweet onion, sliced
- Salt and pepper
- 6 Tblsp. water
- Heat a frying pan over medium high heat. Add the onions and season to taste.
- Cook onions until they turn brown and begin adding water, one tablespoon each time and cook until the water is completely evaporated.

Lemony Asparagus

- 1/3 lb asparagus
- 1 Tblsp. lemon juice
- Sea salt and pepper to taste
- Fill a pot halfway with water and bring to a boil on the stove.
- Rinse and dry asparagus, breaking off the tough part of the stem. Chop remaining stem into 1" lengths. Drop into the boiling water and reduce heat to simmer.
- Cook for 2 minutes and drain. Toss with lemon juice, along with salt and pepper to taste.

Onion Rings

- 1/2 onion, sliced into rings
- 1 melba toast, crumbled
- 1 Tblsp. skim milk
- ¼ tsp. cayenne pepper

- Salt and pepper
- Preheat oven to 350°.
- Mix milk with cayenne and salt to taste. Dip the onion rings into the mixture and then into the melba toast crumbs and place on a baking sheet.
- Bake for 7 minutes, flip and bake another 7 minutes. Line pan with foil to make for easy cleanup.

Baked Onion

- 1 Vidalia onion
- Sea salt
- Pepper
- Preheat oven to 350°.
- Peel onion and add salt and pepper to taste. Wrap in foil and bake for one hour or until tender throughout.

Sauteed Spinach

- ½ bag baby spinach
- 4 Tblsp. chicken broth
- 1 clove garlic, minced
- Saute garlic in 1 Tblsp. broth. When tender, add remaining broth and spinach. Cook until the spinach is soft and remove immediately from the heat.

Easy Tomato Soup

- 1 c. chicken broth
- 1 large tomato
- 1 clove garlic, minced

- ½ tsp. basil
- ½ tsp. onion salt
- ½ tsp. stevia
- Salt and pepper to taste
- Saute the garlic in a hot pan with 1 Tblsp. of broth.
- Blend remaining ingredients in the blender and add to the garlic broth. Bring to a boil and simmer for 10 minutes before serving.

Onion Soup

- 1 onion, sliced
- 3 cloves garlic, minced
- 2 c. beef broth
- 1 tsp. stevia
- Salt and pepper
- Cook onion and garlic in 2 Tblsp. broth for 10 minutes. Add remaining broth and stevia and simmer for 20 minutes. Serve seasoned with salt and pepper.

Spiced Baked Apple

- 1 apple, cut into cubes
- ½ teaspoon cinnamon
- ¼ teaspoon allspice
- Microwave for 1.5 minutes or until tender. Serve hot.

Apple Salad

- 1 apple, cut into thin strips
- 1 teaspoon fresh mint, minced

- 1 tablespoon lemon juice
- Toss all ingredients together in a bowl and serve.

Candy Apples

- 4 apples
- 4 packets stevia
- 1 tsp cinnamon
- 1 tsp. vanilla
- 2 c. water
- Preheat oven to 350°.
- Put apples in a baking dish and add water. Sprinkle apples with stevia and cinnamon. Bake for 1 hour.
- Add vanilla to the water and pour over apples to serve.

Orange Strawberry Smoothie

- 1 c. frozen strawberries
- 1/3 c. fresh orange juice
- ¾ c. ice
- ½ dropper stevia
- Blend until smooth.

Strawberry Sorbet

- 1 c. strawberries, frozen for 1 hour
- Juice of 1 lemon
- Stevia to taste
- Blend all ingredients until smooth. Place in freezer until desired consistency is achieved.

Strawberry "Shortcake"

- 1 strawberry, sliced
- 1 melba toast
- 2 drops vanilla crème stevia
- Place strawberry on top of toast and add stevia. Serve.

Lemon Vinaigrette

- 1 tablespoon lemon juice
- 1 tablespoon balsamic vinegar
- Mix well and use as necessary.

Citrus Vinaigrette

- 2 tablespoon apple cider vinegar
- 1 tablespoon lemon juice
- 1 tablespoon orange juice
- 1/4 tablespoon onion powder
- 1 clove garlic, minced
- Dash of salt
- Mix well and use fresh as a marinade or dressing.

Strawberry Vinegar Dressing

- 5 strawberries
- 1 tablespoon apple cider vinegar
- 1 tablespoon lemon juice
- 1 dropper of Stevia or equivalent of other sweetener
- Dash of salt
- Blend all ingredients in blender until smooth. Serve immediately over vegetables or salad greens.

Spicy Mustard Dressing

- 1 c. apple cider vinegar
- 2 tsp. wasabi powder
- 2 tsp. mustard powder
- Mix all ingredients thoroughly and serve atop salads, fish, etc.

Simple Salsa

- 1 tomato, chopped
- 1 Tbs lemon juice
- 2 cloves garlic, crushed
- 1 tsp onion powder
- 1/4 tsp oregano
- fresh cilantro, chopped
- salt and pepper
- Mix all ingredients together and store in fridge until needed.

Roma Salsa

- 2 Roma tomatoes, chopped
- 2 Tbsp red onion, chopped
- Lemon juice
- Garlic salt
- fresh cilantro, chopped
- Toss tomato and onion together and sprinkle with lemon juice. Stir in garlic salt and add the cilantro. Store in the fridge until needed.

Citrus Tomato Salsa

- 1 large tomato, chopped
- 1 Tblsp. lemon juice
- 1/8 tsp. celery salt
- 1/8 tsp. chili powder
- 3 drops stevia
- 1 tsp. fresh cilantro, minced
- Combine all and refrigerate.

Lunch recipe

Spicy Steak Fajitas

- 1 teaspoon salt
- 1/2 teaspoon ground cumin
- 1/2 teaspoon onion powder
- 1/4 teaspoon garlic powder
- 1/4 cup water
- 3 ½ top round steak.
- 1 green bell pepper- seeded and cut into strips
- 1 medium onion, thinly sliced
- 2 tablespoons fresh lime juice.
- Mix the spices with the water in a Ziploc bag. Add steak, onion and pepper and seal, pressing out most of the air. Knead for a minute to ensure all the ingredients are thoroughly covered and refrigerate for 10-20 minutes.
- Heat a large frying pan over medium heat and add the entire bag of meat and vegetables. Stir from time to time until the steak is cooked to the desired doneness and the vegetables are tender, yet crisp. This should take around 5-7 minutes. Serve hot.

Tomato Burger

- 3 ½ oz. lean ground beef
- 2 large tomato slices
- Pinch garlic powder
- Pinch onion powder
- salt and pepper
- ¼ teaspoon dill

- Pinch coriander
- 1 lettuce leaf
- Mix beef with spices according to preference and pat into a patty. Grill carefully until cooked through. Place patty between two slices of tomato, along with the lettuce. You might want to heat the tomato slices slightly, as well.

Lemon Veal Chops

- 3 ½ oz veal chops
- ½ Tblsp. lemon juice
- Salt and pepper
- Marinate veal in lemon juice in a Ziploc bag for 1 hour.
- Heat frying pan to hot and season veal with salt and pepper. Add to pan and cook for 5 minutes per side.
- Squeeze more lemon juice over meat before serving if desired.

Taco Salad

- 2 cups lettuce, sliced
- 3 ½ oz. ground beef, cooked
- 1 tablespoon cilantro, minced
- salt and pepper
- melba toast, broken up
- 1 tomato, chopped
- Toss all ingredients together and serve cold.

Citrus Beef and Onions

- 3 ½ oz beef

- Juice of ½ lemon
- 3 ½ oz onion, sliced
- Add salt and pepper to the pan, along with onions and a little water. Simmer for 3 minutes.
- Add the meat and lemon juice. Simmer until the meat is cooked to desired doneness. Serve with pan juices.

Beef and Asparagus Soup

- 1 cup beef broth
- 3 ½ oz beef, cooked, cut into pieces
- 1 cup asparagus, chopped
- Mix all ingredients in a pot and heat over medium heat. Simmer until the asparagus is ready.

Beef Chili

- 3 ½ oz lean ground beef
- 1 cup tomatoes, chopped
- ½ cup water
- 1 tablespoon onion, minced
- 2 cloves garlic, crushed and minced
- Pinch of garlic powder
- Pinch of onion powder
- ¼ teaspoon chili powder
- Pinch of oregano
- Cayenne pepper to taste (optional)
- Salt and pepper to taste
- In a small skillet, brown the beef. Add onions, garlic, water and tomatoes and stir. Add spices. Simmer over medium heat until the sauce reduces and thickens.

- Salt and pepper to taste. Serve with tomato slices as a garnish.

Beef Kabobs

- 3 ½ oz beef, cubed
- 1 sweet onion, cut into wedges
- ¼ c. dressing of your choice (see Dressings section)
- Salt and pepper
- Marinate meat and onions with dressing and salt and pepper to taste for at least one hour. Thread onto skewers and grill until meat is tender and done over medium heat.

Lemon Garlic Steak

- 3 ½ oz. steak, cubed
- 1 clove garlic, minced
- 1 lemon, juiced and zested
- Salt and pepper
- Heat frying pan over medium high heat and season steak with salt and pepper to taste.
- Add meat to pan and brown evenly.
- After 5 minutes, add garlic and cook for 1 minute. Add lemon juice and zest and cook another minute. Serve coated in juices.

Tasty Chicken Fajitas

- 1 teaspoon salt
- 1/2 teaspoon ground cumin
- 1/2 teaspoon onion powder
- 1/4 teaspoon garlic powder

- 1/4 cup water
- 6 oz boneless chicken breast in 1/2-inch strips
- 1 green bell pepper – seeded and cut into strips
- 1 medium onion, thinly sliced
- 2 tablespoons fresh lime juice.
- Mix the spices with the water in a Ziploc bag. Add chicken, onion and pepper and seal, pressing out most of the air. Knead for a minute to ensure all the ingredients are thoroughly covered and refrigerate for 10-20 minutes.
- Heat a large frying pan over medium heat and add the entire bag of meat and vegetables. Stir from time to time until the chicken is cooked through and the vegetables are tender, yet crisp. This should take around 5-7 minutes. Serve hot.

Orange Chicken and Broccoli

- 1 chai tea bag
- ¼ cup hot water
- 3 ½ oz chicken, no skin or fat
- 3 ½ oz broccoli, cooked
- 1 orange, peeled and cut into small chunks
- Steep tea bag in hot water for 3 minutes in a sauce pan. Remove tea bag, add chicken pieces and simmer until cooked through.
- Toss the chicken with the broccoli, oranges and the remaining tea. Serve with your choice of spices and salt.

Orange Ginger Chicken

- 3 ½ oz chicken, cut into cubes
- Orange, cut into quarters
- 2 cloves garlic, minced

- 1 Tblsp. fresh ginger, peeled and minced
- ½ tsp. basil
- 1 Tblsp. lemon juice
- Salt and pepper to taste
- Heat a frying pan over medium heat.
- Salt and pepper chicken and add to the pan. Cook for 7-10 minutes. Add garlic and sauté for 1 minute.
- Add lemon juice and squeeze juice from orange sections. Add basil and ginger into the pan, along with peeled orange sections. Cover and simmer for 20 minutes.

Grilled Chicken with Onions and Grapefruit

- 3 ½ oz chicken, no skin or fat
- 3 ½ oz onion, chopped
- ½ grapefruit, peeled and chopped
- Heat onions in 3 tablespoons of water until transparent. Add any herbs you like at this point.
- Add chicken and salt to the pan, as well as additional water if necessary. Cook until chicken is done.
- Toss chicken, grapefruit and onions in a bowl. Add any seasoning you wish.

Chicken Wraps

With these, you can make them ahead and take them with you no matter where you go.

- Sliced, pre-cooked chicken breast
- Leaf lettuce to use as the wrapping shell
- Tomatoes chopped
- Fresh asparagus grilled

- Seasoning for the chicken that you enjoy - garlic, onion and pepper to start
- After broiling the chicken in the oven topped with seasoning, allow to cool slightly. Cut into slices. No serving should be more than 100 grams.

  Take one piece of leaf lettuce and place flat on table. Add half of a serving of the chicken. Add one piece of asparagus and other vegetables you like. Wrap longwise. Repeat with another one.

Cucumber Shrimp Salad

- 100 to 125 grams of shrimp diced
- 1 cup of sliced cucumbers
- White vinegar
- ½ lemon
- Sugar free hot sauce
- Cook 100 to 125 grams of shrimp by steaming it or boiling. Add sugar free hot sauce to the shrimp. Allow to cool completely in the refrigerator for at least one hour.

  Mix in the cucumber, white vinegar to taste and lemon. Serve on Melba toast for enjoy separately.

Buffalo Chicken Salad

Another variety of salad, this one will quench those cravings for something substantial while also giving you some great flavor.

- 100 to 125 grams of chicken breast
- Sugar free buffalo sauce
- Chopped celery, one cup
- ½ cup of chopped onion

- Leaf lettuce to hold chicken salad

Coat chicken in buffalo sauce, ensuring it is sugar free. Add seasoning to taste. Cook chicken breast thoroughly and allow to cook. Baking or broiling is the best method. Allow to cool until you can chop into small pieces. Add to a boil and mix in all other ingredients. Place half of the mixture in a piece of leaf lettuce and wrap up. Repeat for the second half. One serving includes both pieces.

Blackened Chicken Salad

- 100 grams of chicken breast
- ½ teaspoon of garlic powder
- ½ teaspoons of onion powder
- ¼ of a teaspoon of white pepper
- ¼ of a teaspoon of black pepper
- 1/3 of a teaspoon of thyme
- 1 teaspoon of paprika - for more heat, substitute cayenne pepper instead
- ¼ of a teaspoon of ground red pepper
- Leaf lettuce, cabbage or spinach as the bed for the salad

Combine all of the spices into one rub. Rub into the chicken breast thoroughly. Allow to sit for ten minutes to allow for some marinating time. Then, grill the chicken on medium to high heat until fully cooked. Remove and allow to cook. Slice and serve over the top of the lettuce or spinach you select.

Simple Turkey Rollup

A great simple way to have lunch is this recipe. It does not take more than a few minutes to complete!

- 2 slices of lean turkey
- Black pepper
- ¼ teaspoon of smoked paprika
- Strips of celery, cut into long, thin pieces

Place turkey on a surface. Top with pepper and smoked paprika. Place two or three stalks of celery in the middle and roll up.

Veggie Salad

For this salad, create as many varieties as you like by replacing the foods you enjoy that fit into the diet. You can enjoy a range of options.

- 1 cup of spinach
- 1 cup of greens
- ½ cup of chopped onion
- ½ cup of chopped cucumber
- ½ lemon squeezed
- ½ teaspoon freshly ground black pepper
- ½ teaspoon red pepper flakes
- Breadstick on the side
- 100 ounces of chopped turkey

Mix all vegetables together in a large bowl and top with turkey. Add lemon juice as a dressing and top with seasoning. Enjoy the breadstick on the side.

Simple Lettuce Wraps

These are great on the go options, too. Take with you on a hike or to work.

- 3.5 ounces of minced chicken,

- ½ inch of fresh ginger, minced
- 1 clove of garlic, minced
- 1 stalk of green onion, minced
- Whole leaf lettuce
- 1 teaspoon of rice wine vinegar
- 1 cup of vegetable broth from braising

First, braise chicken over medium heat with the ginger, garlic, and onions with vegetable broth until fully cooked.

Then, add rice wine vinegar after dicing chicken. Spoon mixture into leaf lettuce or Bibb lettuce.

Mock Fried Chicken

For those who are craving the types of foods they used to enjoy, try this fake out fried chicken. It could be your go to solution for both lunch and dinner.

Keep in mind that to cut calories even more, you can bake this variety. Frying it will be a bit more realistic in terms of texture but baking it is the healthier option.

- 120 grams of chicken breast
- 1 grissini, crumbled
- ½ teaspoon of paprika
- ½ teaspoon of garlic powder
- ½ teaspoon of black pepper
- ½ teaspoon of dry thyme
- 1 tablespoon of milk
- ½ tablespoon of parmesan cheese
- 2 tablespoons of broth

Heat oven to 350 degrees. Season the chicken with salt and pepper to taste. In one dish, place crumbled grissini and the rest of the seasonings. Coat the chicken with a mixture of the broth and milk. Add a sprinkling of cheese on top. Toss in the grissini crumble mixture. Allow to sit for three to five minutes to rest. Then, place on a non-stick sheet and place in the oven to cook until fully done. The last five minutes, finish under the broiler.

Apple Cider Chicken Salad

This tangy treat is perfect for everything including a great take-to-work meal.

- 125 ounces of chicken breast
- Salad greens of your choice, especially spinach
- 2/3 cup of water
- 1/3 cup of apple cider vinegar
- Salt and pepper to taste

To prepare the chicken, top chicken with salt and pepper to taste. Add smoked paprika, cayenne pepper or other seasonings you enjoy. Broil until cooked and slice. Prepare salad by creating a lettuce bed and topping with chicken. Mix water and vinegar. Top salad with pepper to taste and as much dressing as you would like.

Roasted Vegetables

This recipe calls for asparagus but you can substitute virtually any type of vegetable that you enjoy.

- 100 grams of asparagus with ends trimmed off
- 2 cloves of garlic, minced
- ½ teaspoon of parsley
- ¼ teaspoon of oregano
- Black pepper to taste

On a baking sheet, place asparagus on top of non-stick aluminum foil. Heat oven to 400 degrees. Add seasonings on top. Wrap the asparagus up in the foil to create a small pocket so that the vegetable can steam in the oven. Cook for about 12 to 15 minutes until asparagus are softer.

Spiced Cucumber Salad

This simple dish will give you the flavor you want with plenty of nutrients, too.

- 1 large cucumber
- Sweet and hot flavor seasoning that you prefer without sugar added
- 1 teaspoon of Stevia

Cut up the cucumber into thin slices. Lay them separately in a dish. Pour the sweet and hot seasoning on and allow to sit for three to five minutes before serving. Add Stevia to taste. To make this a complete meal, add a piece of white fish to the marinade as well, without the cucumbers. Cook the fish thoroughly and enjoy with cucumbers.

Spinach, Chicken and Strawberry Salad

This salad is not just good in the summer but all year long.

- 2 cups of spinach
- 100 grams of chicken, broiled, cooled and sliced
- 6 strawberries, cleaned and sliced
- Strawberry vinaigrette made earlier (recipe to follow)

Prepare the strawberry vinaigrette. To do so, combine the following ingredients.

- 3 strawberries

- 1 tablespoon of fresh lemon juice
- 1 tablespoon of apple cider vinegar
- ½ teaspoon of Stevia
- Salt and pepper to taste.

Combine in a food processor. Once combined, store it in an airtight container for up to two weeks in the refrigerator.

To complete the salad, toss the strawberry dressing with the spinach leaves. Add the chicken and fresh cut strawberries. This meal can make a good dinner option, too.

Crab Salad with Honey Mustard Dressing

As long as you can keep it cold, this salad is a great option to take with you throughout the day.

- 2 cups of romaine lettuce
- Lump crab meat that's been cooked, 100 grams
- Melba rounds
- Honey mustard dressing (see recipe below)

For the honey mustard dressing, combine the following ingredients:

- 1/3 cup of apple cider vinegar
- 1 cup of water mixed with 1 cup of Stevia
- 2 ½ tablespoons of your favorite spicy brown mustard (no sugar added)
- ½ teaspoon of salt
- ½ teaspoon of pepper
- ½ teaspoon of garlic powder
- ½ teaspoon of onion powder.

Shake well and store in an airtight container for up to two weeks in the refrigerator.

To complete the salad, simply combine the romaine lettuce with crab meat. Then, top with about two tablespoons of the honey mustard dressing. Serve on Melba rounds.

Meat and Tomato Sauce

Enjoy this on top of a bed of greens if you like or on Melba toast.

- 1 large tomato
- 100 grams of lean ground beef (you can also substitute white fish, shrimp or chicken)
- ¼ teaspoon of garlic salt
- ¼ teaspoon of onion salt
- ½ teaspoon of Italian seasoning

Cut the tomato into small chunks. Put into a saucepan and allow it to breakdown for about five minutes. Use a fork to smash the pieces of tomato to encourage it to become more of a thick sauce. Add in the seasonings and allow to cook. In a frying pan, add meat and brown thoroughly. Once browned, add to the sauce and allow to simmer for two to three minutes until it becomes one sauce. Serve on toast.

Dinner

Lemon Basil Chicken

- 3 ½ oz chicken, no skin or fat
- 3 ½ oz tomatoes chopped
- Juice of ½ lemon
- Basil, fresh or dried
- Place chicken in a frying pan, along with the lemon juice and additional water if required. Cook over medium heat for 2-4 minutes. Add tomatoes and basil, reducing heat to low. Simmer until the chicken is cooked through, turning halfway through.
- Serve with the self-made sauce over lettuce.

Chicken Cabbage Wraps

- 3.5 ounces chicken
- 2 medium red cabbage leaves
- 1 garlic clove, minced
- 3 tablespoons balsamic vinegar
- 1/4 teaspoons onion powder
- 1/4 tablespoon sea salt
- 1/4 tablespoon pepper
- 1 tablespoon fresh ginger, finely grated
- Mix ginger, garlic, salt, onion powder and vinegar with pepper. Toss chicken in the mixture and cook over medium-high heat until done, turning once. Add the cabbage leaves and heat until soft and barely cooked.

- Lay out the cabbage leaves and place half the chicken mixture on each. Roll tightly and serve.

Basil Chicken

- Cooking spray
- 1/2 cup onion, chopped fine
- 1 clove garlic, minced
- 2 ½ cup tomatoes, chopped
- 2 c. Boneless chicken breast halves, cut into chunks
- 1/4 cup fresh basil, minced
- 1/2 tsp. salt
- 1/8 tsp. hot pepper sauce
- Lightly spray a large frying pan with cooking spray and heat onions and garlic over medium-high heat. Add chicken and remaining ingredients. Reduce the heat to medium and cover the frying pan.
- Simmer mixture, stirring, until the chicken is cooked through and the tomatoes soft.

Fried Chicken

- 1 chicken breast
- 1 Tblsp. milk
- 1 crushed melba toast
- Salt and pepper
- Dip chicken in milk and cover with melba crumbs. Cook in a non-stick pan over medium heat until cooked through. Salt and pepper to taste.

Creole Baked Chicken

- 4 chicken breasts
- 1 onion, chopped
- 2 cloves garlic, minced
- Creole seasoning
- Preheat oven to 350°.
- Rub chicken breasts with creole seasoning. Sprinkle with onion and garlic and cover with foil. Bake for 40 minutes.

Blackened Baked Chicken

- 1/2 tsp. paprika
- 1/8 tsp. salt
- 1/4 tsp. cayenne pepper
- 1/4 tsp. ground cumin
- 1/4 tsp. dried thyme
- 1/8 tsp. ground white pepper
- 1/8 tsp. onion powder
- 2 skinless, boneless chicken breast halves
- Preheat oven to 350° and grease a cookie sheet.
- In a bowl, toss together all the spices. Use cooking spray to oil the chicken breasts on both sides, then coat with spices.
- Cook in a hot frying pan one minute per side and place breasts on the cookie sheet. Bake until juices are clear when the breasts are poked with a knife.

Chicken Chili

- 3 ½ oz ground beef
- 1 c. cabbage, grated
- 2 Roma tomatoes, chopped

- 2 c. water
- 2 cloves garlic, minced
- 1/2 tsp. cumin
- 1/2 tsp. chili powder
- 1/2 tsp. oregano
- 1/2 tsp. thyme
- Salt and pepper to taste
- Cook meat and garlic in a large frying pan until meat is browned. Add water and spices and bring to a boil.
- Add cabbage and cook until tender over medium high heat. Stir in the tomato and simmer for 5-10 minutes. Add salt to taste.

Chicken Adobo

- 1 chicken breast
- ¼ c. apple cider vinegar
- ¼ c. low sodium soy sauce
- ¼ onion, diced
- 1 garlic clove, minced
- 1 bay leaf
- ¼ tsp. ginger
- Spray a frying pan with cooking spray and cook onion and garlic over medium low heat until tender.
- Add everything but the chicken and cook until bubbles form. Add the chicken and simmer until done, turning occasionally, for about 10 minutes.

Cajun Chicken

- 2 chicken breasts
- 2 tsp. water

- 1/8 tsp each garlic powder, pepper, salt, onion powder
- Mix spices with water to form a paste. Rub onto the chicken and refrigerate for 1 hour. Grill over medium heat until done.

Strawberry Chicken Salad

- 3 1/2 oz. chicken
- ¼ teaspoon garlic powder
- ¼ teaspoon oregano powder
- Spinach leaves, torn
- Strawberry Vinegar Dressing (see Sauce and Dressings section)
- Sprinkle chicken with the garlic and oregano and cook in a hot frying pan until done. Cut into slices and toss with dressing and spinach.

Jerk Turkey Salad

- 3 ½ oz of turkey breast
- 1 tablespoon Caribbean jerk seasoning
- ½ cucumber, peeled and sliced
- 2 oz fresh pineapple, chopped
- 2 oz strawberries
- ¼ cup celery, sliced
- 2 slices of green onion
- ¼ cup lime juice
- Salt and cumin to taste.
- Rub jerk seasoning into the turkey breast. Preheat grill or frying pan to medium heat and place the turkey on it. Cook until turkey is cooked through. Remove from heat and allow to cool.

- Cut turkey into small pieces and toss with remaining ingredients, adding salt and cumin to taste.

Spicy Crab with Cucumber

- 3 ½ oz crab meat
- 1 tsp. lime juice
- 1 tsp. water
- 1 tsp. green onions, chopped
- ½ tsp. dry mustard powder
- Red pepper flakes to taste
- ½ cucumber, sliced
- Mix crab and the spices, along with the water and lime juice. Top slices of cucumber with the mixture and serve.

Grilled Shrimp in Marinade

- ¼ cup chopped cilantro
- Juice of 1 lemon
- 3 cloves garlic, minced
- 1 teaspoon salt
- 1 teaspoon cumin
- 6 oz. large cooked shrimp
- Toss all ingredients in a Ziploc bag and refrigerate for up to an hour.
- Preheat grill on medium and grill the shrimp until opaque. This takes about 5 minutes per side.

Seafood Gumbo

- 3 ½ oz any seafood

- 1 garlic clove, minced
- 2 Roma tomatoes, chopped
- ¼ tsp. onion salt
- ¼ tsp. creole seasoning
- 1/8 tsp. garlic powder
- 1/8 tsp. cayenne pepper
- 1 packet stevia
- Saute garlic and seafood for 1 minute over high heat. Add remaining ingredients and reduce heat to simmer. Cook for 15 minutes.

Fish Tacos

- 3 ½ oz. white fish, cut into pieces
- pinch chili powder
- pinch garlic powder
- pinch onion powder
- salt and pepper
- 1-2 large cabbage leaves
- melba toast
- Toss fish and spices together in a frying pan and cook with a little water until done. Drain the fish.
- Microwave the cabbage for 30 seconds to make the leaves soft. Split the fish mixture in half and spread on each leaf. Sprinkle the melba toast crumbles over the fish, roll it all up and serve.

Lime Whitefish

- 3 ½ oz whitefish
- 1 ½ tsp. liquid aminos
- ¼ tsp. fresh ginger, grated

- Lime, cut into wedges
- Salt and pepper
- Squeeze half the lime into a bowl and add ginger and liquid aminos. Stir well.
- Marinate the fish for 20 minutes in the solution, coating thoroughly.
- Salt and pepper to taste and cook with marinade in a hot frying pan, 3-5 minutes per side.

Grilled Scallops

- ¼ lb. jumbo scallops
- 2 tsp. Cajun seasoning
- Rinse and dry scallops. Place on skewers and season on both sides.
- Heat a pan to medium high heat and add scallop skewers. Cook for 3-4 minutes per side.

Fried Fish

- 3 ½ oz fish
- 1 Tblsp. milk
- 1 crushed melba toast
- Salt and pepper
- Dip fish in milk and cover with melba crumbs. Cook in a non-stick pan over medium heat until cooked through. Salt and pepper to taste.

Herbed Fish with Broccoli

- 3 ½ oz white fish

- 3 ½ oz broccoli, chopped
- 1 Tomato, peeled and chopped
- Basil, thyme, oregano, dried or fresh
- Juice of ½ lemon
- Heat a frying pan over medium heat and add herbs and fish. Drizzle lemon juice over the fish and add broccoli and tomatoes. If needed, add a small amount of water.
- Simmer until the fish is cooked through. Serve with the pan juices.

Lemon Tilapia with Grapefruit

- 3 ½ oz Tilapia fish
- Juice of half a lemon
- Salt, pepper and dill
- ½ grapefruit sliced in small pieces
- Heat frying pan to medium heat and add the fish. Drizzle with lemon juice and add slices of lemon around the fish. Sprinkle with salt, pepper and dill as you like.
- Cook until the fish is done and serve with grapefruit pieces.

Ceviche

- 3 ½ oz. white fish or shrimp, cooked and chilled
- 3 tablespoons lemon or lime juice
- Diced tomatoes
- 1 tablespoon chopped onion
- 1 clove garlic crushed and minced
- Fresh chopped cilantro
- Dash hot sauce
- Salt and pepper to taste

- Chop the fish or shrimp into small chunks. Add remaining ingredients and toss. Chill for 1 hour before serving.

Quick and Easy Baked Fish

- 3 ½ oz fish
- Juice of ½ lemon
- Salt, pepper and dill
- Preheat oven to 350°.
- Lay fish on a large piece of aluminum foil. Add lemon juice and slice the lemon up. Place slices around the fish and season with dill, salt and pepper. Fold the foil up to form a packet and seal the fish in.
- Bake until done, about 10-15 minutes.

Lobster with Onions

- 3 ½ oz Lobster pieces
- Juice of ½ lemon
- Salt, pepper and dill
- 3 ½ oz onion slices
- mustard and seasonings
- Heat onion and 2 tablespoons of water in a frying pan over medium heat until the onion is tender. Add lobster, lemon juice and seasonings to taste. Cook until the fish is done.
- Add mustard to taste and serve.

Conclusion

Thank you again for downloading this book!

I hope this book was able to help you to understand the HCG diet plan and prepare you for your journey. The diet plan may be a tough process that you will have to go through but the intrinsic rewards are endless. Every time you feel that you have to give up, just imagine the the person you will be after the diet plan. That is the person you are giving up.

Finally, if you enjoyed this book, then I'd like to ask you for a favor, would you be kind enough to leave a review for this book on Amazon? It'd be greatly appreciated!

Click here to leave a review for this book on Amazon!

Thank you and good luck!

Made in the USA
San Bernardino, CA
24 April 2019